INFLAMMATION

ANAPHYLAXIS

What is it?	Symptoms	Treatment
Anaphylaxis is a severe and potentially life threatening allergic reaction which can happen very suddenly when exposed to allergen. This causes the immune system to release chemicals which reduce blood pressure suddenly and narrow the airway. If left untreated it can be fatal	<ul><li>Hives</li><li>Itching skin</li><li>Flushed or pale</li><li>Hypotension</li><li>Swollen tongue</li><li>Wheezy</li><li>Weak rapid pulse</li><li>Nausea/vomiting</li><li>Diarrhoea</li><li>Dizziness/fainting</li></ul>	<ul><li>I in 1000 adrenaline</li><li>Chlorphemamine</li><li>Hydrocortisone</li><li>Make sure you check doses will change depending on age</li><li>High flow Oxygen—Salbutamol may also help with the wheeze and to open up the airway</li><li>They may also need fluids if hypotensive</li></ul>

What is it?	Symptoms	Treatment
• Sepsis is a multi system response to the invasion of a pathogen, potential pathogen or micro-organism. • Small amounts of cytokines are released into circulation, leading to inflammatory mediator cells to get involved. • Sepsis is a failure to control the inflammatory cascade which leads to organ injury and dysfunction	• Lethargy • Fever • Headaches • New onset confusion • Shortness of breath • Diarrhoea • Vomiting • Hypotension	Pre hospital treatment • Oxygen if need to maintain sats between 94-98% • IV fluids if hypotensive • Pre alert into hospital • Work out a NEWS 2 score Sepsis 6 • Give oxygen to keep sats above 94% • Take blood cultures • Give IV antibiotics • Give a fluid challenge • Measure lactate • Measure urine output

NEUROGENIC SHOCK

What is it?	Symptoms	Treatment

• Is a life-threatening condition caused by irregular blood circulation in the body
• It can cause the blood pressure to drop drastically and suddenly which can cause irreversible organ damage or even death
	• Dizziness
	• Nausea
	• Vomiting
	• Blank stares
	• Fainting
	• Increased sweating
	• Anxiety
	• Pale skin
	• Difficulty breathing
	• Chest pain
	• Weakness
	• Bradycardia
	• Faint pulse
	• Hypothermia
	• Cyanosis
		• Medications such as
		  ○ Norepinephrine
		  ○ Epinephrine
		  ○ Dopamine
		  ○ Vasopressin

HYPOVOLAEMIC SHOCK

What is it?	Symptoms	Treatment
• Is a life-threatening condition that results in the loss of more than 20% of the body's fluid • It is the most common cause of shock • The severe fluid loss means that the heart cannot pump sufficient amount of blood to the body which can lead to organ failure so immediate medical intervention is needed	• Headache • Fatigue • Nausea • Sweating • Dizziness • Cold clammy skin • Pale skin • Rapid breathing • Tachycardia • Reduced urination • Confusion • Weakness • Weak pulse • Cyanosis • Light-headedness • Loss of consciousness	• Blood transfusion • Medication

OBSTRUCTIVE SHOCK

What is it?	Symptoms	Treatment
• Is a form of shock that is associated with a physical blockage in the great vessels of the body or the heart causing a lack of perfusion • It is very similar to cardiogenic shock and maybe diagnosed together	• Rapid breathing • Severe shortness of breath • Tachycardia • Loss of consciousness • Weak pulse • Hypotension • Sweating • Pale skin • Cold hands and or feet • Reduced urination	• Treat the cause

CARDIOGENIC SHOCK

What is it?	Symptoms	Treatment

• Is a life-threatening condition where the heart suddenly cannot pump enough blood to meet the needs of the body
• It is most commonly caused by having a heart attack however not everyone has a heart attack will have cardiogenic shock
• Due to the seriousness of the condition if not treated immediately they will die, it has a mortality rate of around 50%
	• Rapid breathing
	• Severe shortness of breath
	• Tachycardia
	• Loss of consciousness
	• Weak pulse
	• Hypotension
	• Sweating
	• Pale skin
	• Cold hands and or feet
	• Reduced urination
		• Emergency life support
		• Medications
		  ○ Vasopressin
		  ○ Inotropic agents
		  ○ Aspirin
		  ○ Antiplatelets
		  ○ Blood thinners
		• Surgery
		  ○ ECMO
		  ○ Angioplasty
		  ○ Stents
		  ○ Balloon pump
		  ○ VAD
		  ○ Heart transplant
		  ○ Coronary artery bypass surgery
		  ○ Surgery to repair the damaged or injury to the heart

CARDIOVASCULAR

What is it?	Symptoms	Treatment

Is chest pain caused by decreased coronary blood-flow and increased myocardial oxygen consumption which leads to a decrease in the oxygen supply/ demand ratio and myocardial hypoxia	• Nausea
	• Shortness of breath
	• Abdominal pain
	• Discomfort in the neck, jaw or back
	• Stabbing pain instead of chest pressure
	• Dizziness
	• Fatigue
	• Shortness of breath
	• Sweating
		• Medications
		  ○ Nitrates
		  ○ Aspirin
		  ○ Anticoagulants
		  ○ Beta blockers
		  ○ Statins
		  ○ Calcium channel blockers
		  ○ Blood pressure medications
		  ○ GTN
		• Procedures
		  ○ Angioplasty
		  ○ Stenting
		  ○ ECP
		  ○ Coronary artery bypass surgery

CORONARY ARTERY DISEASE

What is it?	Symptoms	Treatment

• This is where the coronary arteries become diseased or damaged - This is usually cause dry plaques, containing cholesterol deposit on the coronary artery or the inflammation of the coronary artery disease
• The build-up of plaque and inflammation cause the arteries to narrow causing which will cause symptoms
• A complete blockage would cause an MI
	• Chest pain
	• Shortness of breath
	• MI
		• Lifestyle changes
		  ○ Quit smoking
		  ○ Healthy eating
		  ○ Regular exercise
		  ○ Loss of excess weight
		  ○ Reduce stress
		• Drugs
		  ○ Aspirin
		  ○ Beta blockers
		  ○ Nitroglycerin
		  ○ ACE inhibitors
		  ○ Calcium channel blockers
		• Procedures
		  ○ Angioplasty and stent placement
		  ○ Coronary artery bypass surgery

What is it?	Symptoms	Treatment

• Also known as congestive heart failure
• It occurs when the heart muscle does not pump blood as well as it should
• The heart may not provide tissues with adequate blood for metabolic needs, and cardiac-related elevation of pulmonary or systemic venous pressures may result in organ congestion.
	• Fatigue and weakness
	• Oedema in your legs, ankles and feet
	• Rapid or irregular heartbeat
	• Reduced ability to exercise
	• Persistent cough or wheezing with white or pink blood-tinged phlegm
	• Increased need to urinate at night
	• Swelling of your abdomen (ascites)
	• Very rapid weight gain from fluid retention
	• Lack of appetite and nausea
	• Difficulty concentrating or decreased alertness
	• Sudden, severe shortness of breath and coughing up pink, foamy mucus
	• Chest pain if your heart failure is caused by a heart
		• Medications
		  ○ Digoxin
		  ○ Inotropes
		  ○ Aldosterone antagonists
		  ○ Diuretics
		  ○ Beta blockers
		  ○ Angiotensin 2 receptor blockers
		  ○ ACE inhibitors
		• Surgery
		  ○ Heart transplant
		  ○ LVADs
		  ○ Cardiac resynchronisation therapy
		  ○ ICDs
		  ○ Heart valve repair or replacement
		  ○ Coronary bypass surgery

DEEP VEIN THROMBOSIS

What is it?	Symptoms	Treatment

• DVTs are thrombus (clots) within the deep veins of the deep veins of the legs which left untreated are the primary cause of pulmonary embolism
• DVTs come from impaired venous return which can be caused by injury or dysfunction or by hypercoagulability
• Many DVTs are asymptomatic or they will cause pain and swelling the affected leg
	• Leg swelling
	• Leg pain
	• Leg cramping
	• Change in colour on the leg such as redness or purple
	• A warm feeling in the leg
	• Serious symptoms when it travels to the lungs where it PE is life threatening
	  ○ Sudden shortness of breath
	  ○ Chest pain
	  ○ Lightheadedness
	  ○ Dizziness
	  ○ Fainting
	  ○ Rapid pulse
	  ○ Rapid breathing
	  ○ Coughing up blood
		• Blood thinners
		• Thrombolytics
		• Filters
		• Compression stockings

What is it?	Symptoms	Treatment
• ACS is a range of conditions that are associated with a sudden and reduced blood flow to the heart • These conditions include heart attacks and angina • It will often cause chest pain or discomfort and is a medical emergency that needs treatment to restore blood flow, treat complications and prevent future problems	• Chest pain • Pain spreading from the chest to the shoulders, arms, neck and jaw • Nausea/vomiting • Indigestion • Shortness of breath • Sudden sweating • Pallor • Dizziness/ fainting • Unexplained fatigue • Feeling restless and apprehensive	• 12 lead ECG • GTN • Aspirin • Transport to hospital for troponin levels • If ECG shows MI then follow the STEMI/NSTEMI care bundle

MYOCARDIAL INFARCTION

What is it?	Symptoms	Treatment

A MI occurs when the flow of blood to the heart is blocked either fully or partially. The blockage can be caused by a buildup of fat or cholesterol which forms plaques in the coronary arteries. Sometime the plaque can rupture and form a clot that blocks this blockage causes the an interruption in the blood flow which will damage the heart muscle and even destroy part of the heart muscle.	• Jaw pain
	• Neck pain
	• Pain down the left arm
	• Chest pain
	• Nausea
	• Indigestion
	• Heartburn
	• Abdominal pain
	• Shortness of breath
	• Cold sweat
	• Fatigue
	• Lightheadedness
	• Sudden dizziness
		• STEMI
		  ○ GTN
		  ○ Aspirin
		  ○ Morphine for pain if needed
		  ○ Hospital transfer for PPCI
		• NSTEMI
		  ○ GTN
		  ○ Aspirin
		  ○ Morphine for pain if needed
		  ○ Hospital transfer

What is it?	Symptoms	Treatment

An abnormal weakening in the lining of an artery wall which causes a buttoning effect resulting and is usually asymptomatic for a long period of time.	• Sudden extreme severe headache
	• Nausea and vomiting
	• Blurred or double vision
	• Sensitivity to light
	• Seizure
	• A drooping eyelid
	• Loss of consciousness
	• Confusion
	• Lower back pain
	• Pulsating mass
	• Fatigue
	• Hypotension
	• Tachycardia
		• Pre hospital
		  ○ Treat the symptoms such as pain and hypotension
		  ○ Do they need a rapid transfer
		  ○ If the aneurysm ruptured do they meet TXA criteria
		• Hospital
		  ○ Observation of the aneurysm if rupture risk is low
		  ○ Surgery

ENDOCARDITIS

What is it?	Symptoms	Treatment
Endocarditis is a life-threatening inflammation or the endocardium the inner layer of the heart including the chambers and valves	<ul><li>Aching joints and muscles</li><li>Chest pain on inhalation and exhalation</li><li>Fatigue</li><li>Fever</li><li>Night sweats</li><li>Shortness of breath</li><li>Swelling of the feet, legs or abdomen</li><li>New or changed heart murmur</li></ul>	<ul><li>Medications</li><li>Surgery to fix the damage</li></ul>

MYOCARDITIS

What is it?	Symptoms	Treatment
• Is the inflammation of the myocardium the muscle of the heart that is not secondary to ischemic events or cardiac rejection in the setting of transplantation • The presence of myocyte necrosis is required for some types of myocarditis.	• Chest pain • Rapid or abnormal heart rhythms • Shortness of breath at rest as well as during • exercise • Fluid retention with swelling in the legs, ankles • and feet • Fatigue • Fever and chills • Headaches • Muscle aches • Joint pain • Sore throat • Diarrhoea • Cough	• Corticosteroid therapy • Cardiac medications such as beta-blockers and ACE inhibitors • Antibiotic therapy • Diuretic therapy to treat fluid overload • Fluid restriction • Low- salt diet • Rest

PERICARDITIS

What is it?	Symptoms	Treatment

• Is swelling and irritation to the pericardium
• Pain is caused when the irritated layers of the pericardium rubs against each other
	• Pain in the chest
	• Left sided shoulder pain
	• Neck pain
	• Pain that gets worse when they cough, lie down or take a deep breath
	• Abdominal or leg swelling
	• Cough
	• Fatigue
	• Fever
	• Heart palpitation
	• Shortness of breath
		• Medications
		  ○ Pain relief
		  ○ Corticosteroids
		• Surgeries/ procedures
		  ○ Pericardiocentesis
		  ○ Pericardiectomy

COMPARTMENT SYNDROME

What is it?	Acute compartment syndrome	Chronic compartment syndrome

• It is a painful and potentially serious condition caused by bleeding or swelling within an enclosed bundle of muscles known as the muscle compartment
• It occurs when pressure within the compartment increases restricting blood flow to the area and potentially damaging the muscle and nearby nerves
• It will usually occur in the legs, feet, arms, or hands however it can happen wherever there is an enclosed compartment in the body
	• Happens suddenly, usually after severe injury or fracture
	• This is a medical emergency and requires urgent treatment
	• It can lead to permanent muscle damage if not treated quickly
	• Signs and Symptoms
	  ○ Intense pain
	  ○ Tenderness in affected area
	  ○ Tightness of the muscle
	  ○ Tingling/burning sensation
	  ○ Numbness/ Weakness
	• Causes
	  ○ Broken bones
	  ○ Crush injuries
	  ○ Constrictive items which don't allow room for swelling
	  ○ Burns
	  ○ Surgery to repair a damaged or block blood vessel
	• Treatment
	  ○ Emergency Fasciotomy
		• Happens gradually, usually during and immediately after repetitive exercise
		• Normally passes soon after stopping the activity
		• It is not a medical emergency and does not cause permanent damage
		• Signs and Symptoms
		  ○ Cramping pain during exercise
		  ○ Swelling to visible budging muscle
		  ○ Tingling sensation
		  ○ The affected area may turn pale and cold
		  ○ Difficulty moving the affected area in serve cases
		• Causes
		  ○ The exact cause is unknown however the theory is that it is caused by temporary swelling of a muscle during exercise which affects the blood supply to a whole group of muscles
		• Treatment
		  ○ Physiotherapy
		  ○ NSAIDs
		  ○ Orthotics

RESPIRATORY

What is it?	Symptoms	Treatment

• Is a condition in which your airways narrow and swells and produce extra mucus.
• Causes variable and recurrent episodes of wheezing, breathlessness, chest tightness and a cough.
• Associated with widespread but variable airflow obstruction that is often reversible
	• Shortness of breath
	• Chest tightness or pain
	• Wheezing when exhaling
	• Trouble sleeping caused by shortness of breath, coughing or wheezing.
	• Being too breathless to eat, speak or sleep
	• Breathing faster
	• A fast heartbeat
	• Drowsiness, confusion, exhaustion or dizziness
	• Blue lips or fingers
	• Fainting
		• Mild/moderate
		  o If O2 levels are normal encourage patient to use their own inhaler if they don't think about giving salbutamol nebuliser
		• Acute severe
		  o Salbutamol nebuliser
		  o Ipratropium bromide nebuliser
		  o Hydrocortisone-IM/IV
		• Life threatening
		  o Salbutamol nebuliser
		  o Ipratropium bromide nebuliser
		  o Hydrocortisone-IM/IV
		  o Adrenaline 1 in 1000- IM
		  o High flow oxygen

PULMONARY EMBOLISM

What is it?	Symptoms	Treatment

• A pulmonary embolism is a blockage in one or more pulmonary arteries
• Most pulmonary is caused by a DVT or in rare occasions a deep vein thrombosis travelling to the lungs
	• Shortness of breath
	• Chest pain
	• Cough
	• Fever
	• Clammy
	• Cyanosis
	• Dizziness
	• Palpation
	• Tachycardia
		• Hospital
		  ○ Anticoagulants
		  ○ Thrombolytics
		• Prehospital
		  ○ Maintain SPO2 levels
		  ○ Treat the pain
		  ○ Transport to nearest Emergency department

HYPOXIA

What is it?	Symptoms	Treatment
Is a condition in which the body or a specific area of the body area of the body is deprived of oxygen	• Changes of colour of the skin • Confusion • Cough • Tachycardia • Rapid breathing • Shortness of breath • Bradycardia • Sweating • Wheezing	• Oxygen therapy • Medications

CHRONIC OBSTRUCTIVE PULMONARY DISEASE

What is it?	Symptoms	Treatment

Is characterised by airflow obstruction that is caused by chronic bronchitis or emphysema, the obstruction is caused by inflammation which changes the structural function of the lungs which makes it harder to expel CO2. The air will become trapped causing the chest to hyper-expand and become a barrel shape which prevents more air from being expired. Because of this the patient will retain CO2 and become hypoxia. This pressure can damage the alveoli further causing a snowball effect of decreasing function	• Breathlessness
	• Chronic cough
	• Regular sputum production
	• Frequent bronchitis especially in the winter
	• Wheeze
	• Chest tightness
	• Lack of energy
	• Unintended weight loss
	• Swelling in the feet, ankles and legs
		• Assess ABCD's
		• Position the patient in the most comfortable position that also easies respiration
		• Consider ventilation
		• Ask patient I'd they're have an individualised treatment plan
		• Assess if this is a acute exacerbation of COPD
		• Do they need a bronchodilator such as nebuliser salbutamol or ipratropium bromide
		• Respiratory rate
		• Oxygen saturation
		• They could be between 88-92% with COPD
		• Do they need oxygen
		  ○ Caution- hypoxia drive
		• Pulse
		• Blood pressure
		  ○ If low do they need fluids
		• Blood glucose level
		  ○ Are they hypo/hyperglycaemic
		• Temperature
		• NEWS2 - Could they be septic
		• ECG if required
		• Assess if patient is in pain
		  ○ Do they need any analgesia
		  ○ Complete documentation
		• Transfer
		• Do they need to go to A&E or is there an alternative pathway for them or arrange a follow up

ACUTE BRONCHITIS

What is it?	Symptoms	Treatment
Is inflammation of the lining of the bronchi often developed during a cold or other respiratory illness	• Fatigue • Shortness of breath • Cough • Fever • Chest discomfort • Sputum that can be clear, which, yellow or green	• Cough medicine

PNEUMONIA

What is it?	Symptoms	Treatment
• Is an infection that inflames the alveoli in one or both lungs • It causes the alveoli to fill with fluid causing someone to cough with phlegm	• Chest pain when you breathe or cough • Confusion or changes in mental awareness • Cough, which may produce phlegm • Fatigue • Fever • Lower than normal body temperature • Nausea & vomiting • Diarrhoea • Shortness of breath	• Antibiotics • Cough medicine • Antipyretics • Analgesic

NEUROLOGICAL

MENINGITIS

What is it?	Symptoms	Pre hospital treatment
• Acute inflammation of the Meninges caused by either viral or bacterial infection • The causative agent enters the CSF and spreads throughout the subarachnoid space • Resulting inflammation, exudates production and tissue damage to the brain result in pyrexia and increased ICP	• Petechial rash • Altered mental state • Cold hands and feet • Extremity pain • Fever • Headache • Neck stiffness • Mottled skin • Delayed capillary refill	• ABCDE approach • High oxygen SpO2 >95% (except COPD) • Assist ventilations if SpO2 30 or chest expansion inadequate • Correct A and B problems on scene, Do Not delay transport • Administer benzylpenicillin in transit (slow IV or IM injection) • Correct hypoglycaemia • Consider IV fluid replacement • Ongoing assessment and management of ABCs in transit – be aware of rapid deterioration in condition

SEIZURES

What is it?	Symptoms	Treatment

A seizure is a sudden, uncontrolled electrical disturbance in the brain, it can cause changes in behaviour, movements, feelings, and levels of consciousness	• Temporary confusion
	• Starring spells
	• Uncontrolled jerking of the limbs
	• Loss of consciousness
	• Loss of awareness
	• Cognitive or emotional symptoms
	  ○ Deja V1
	  ○ Fear
	  ○ Anxiety
		• Medications, pre hospital you can give diazepam or midazolam depending on the trust
		• Diet control
		• Surgery
		• Electrical stimulation

SYNCOPE

What is it?	Symptoms	Treatment
A syncope also known as a faint which is a transient loss of consciousness usually caused by insufficient blood flow to the vein	• Dizziness • Tinnitus • Weakness • Nausea, vomiting • Blurred vision • Paleness • Headache • Incontinence • Sensation that the room is moving • Tingling and numbness of finger tips and around the lips • Bluish cast to the skin • Shortness of breath	• Treat the cause • Raise the legs- increases venous return • Promote fluids

What is it?	Symptoms	Treatment

• A stroke occurs when the blood supply to a part of a brain is cut off or reduced. This prevents the brain tissue from getting the oxygen and nutrients causing the brain cells to die within minutes
 	
• A TIA is a temporary period of symptoms similar to those of a stroke. The symptoms last anywhere from a few minutes to 24 hours.
	• Hemiparesis or hemiplegia
	• Numbness
	• Confusion or coma
	• Convulsions
	• Incontinence
	• Slurred speech
	• Facial weakness
	• Headache
	• Nausea and vomiting
	• Convulsion
	• Loss of consciousness
	• As the haemorrhage expands, ICP rises causing coma and Cushing reflexes
	• Sudden severe headache
		• Check ABCD's
		• FAST test
		• Assess the Patients GCS
		• Take a set of physiological observations
		  ○ Pulse
		  ○ Resp rate
		  ○ Oxygen Sats
		    ■ Do they need Oxygen
		  ○ Blood pressure
		    ■ Consider fluids if it's low
		  ○ Blood glucose
		    ■ Hypoglycaemia can mimic a stroke
		      • Give Glucose if they are hypoglycaemic
		  ○ Temperature
		  ○ Work out NEWS2 score
		• ECG
		• Assess Patients Pain
		• Transfer to Hospital - Ideally a Stroke unit - Pre alert so hospital knows they are coming - Documentation
		Hospital Treatment
		• Ischemic stroke
		  ○ IV thrombolysis
		  ○ Emergency endovascular procedures
		• Haemorrhagic stroke
		  ○ Emergency measures
		  ○ Surgery
		  ○ Rehabilitation

Types	Symptoms	Treatment
Tension headache	Usually dull, persistent, non-throbbing	
Sinus headache	• Pain, pressure and fullness in the cheeks, brow or forehead. • Worsening pain if you bend forward or lie down. • Stuffy nose. • Fatigue. • Achy feeling in the upper teeth.	• Drink plenty of water • Get plenty of rest • Try to relax • Take over the counter painkillers such as paracetamol or ibuprofen

Migraines	• The main symptom of a migraine is usually an intense headache on 1 side of the head.
	• Other symptoms commonly associated with a migraine include:
	  ○ feeling sick.
	  ○ being sick.
	  ○ increased sensitivity to light and sound	

Cluster headahes	Occurs in bursts, often during sleep - Severe pain in and around one eye	

ABDOMINAL

What is it?	Symptoms	Treatment
<ul><li>Is an umbrella term used to describe disorders that involve chronic inflammation of the digestive tract</li><li>The main conditions are</li><ul><li>Ulcerative colitis</li><ul><li>Is a condition which involves inflammation and ulcers along the superficial lining of the colon and rectum</li></ul><li>Crohn's disease</li><ul><li>Is inflammation of the digestive tract but can involve the deeper layers of the digestive tract</li></ul></ul></ul>	<ul><li>Diarrhoea</li><li>Fatigue</li><li>Abdominal pain</li><li>Abdominal cramping</li><li>Blood in stool</li><li>Reduced appetite</li><li>Unintended weight loss</li></ul>	<ul><li>Anti-inflammatory drugs</li><li>Immune system suppressors</li><li>Biologics</li><li>Antibiotics</li><li>Nutritional support</li><li>Surgery</li></ul>

PANCREATITIS

What is it?	Symptoms	Treatment
Is the inflammation in the pancreas	<ul><li>Upper abdominal</li><li>Fever</li><li>Pain worse after eating</li><li>Tachycardia</li><li>Nausea/ vomiting</li><li>Loss of weight without trying</li><li>Oily, smelly stool</li></ul>	<ul><li>Fasting</li><li>IV fluids</li><li>Analgesia</li><li>Surgery</li></ul>

APPENDICITIS

What is it?	Symptoms	Treatment
Is the inflammation of the appendix caused by an obstruction of the appendix lumen by faecal matters foreign body or worms. This leads to distension, bacterial overgrowth, and inflammation. If left untreated necrosis, gangrene and perforation will occur.	<ul><li>Sudden abdominal pain in the iliac fossa</li><li>Nausea/vomiting</li><li>Loss of appetite</li><li>Fever</li><li>Constipation</li><li>Diarrhoea</li><li>Abdominal bloating</li><li>Flatulence</li></ul>	<ul><li>Surgery to remove appendix</li><li>Antibiotics</li><li>Appropriate pain relief</li></ul>

What is it?	Symptoms	Treatment
• Chronic constipation is infrequent bowel movement or difficultly passing of stool that can persists for several weeks or longer. • Constipation is described as having fewer than three bowel movements a week	• Passing fewer than 3 stools a week • Lumpy or hard stools • Straining to have a bowel movement • Feeling as though there's a blockage in the rectum • Can not fully empty rectum • Abdominal distension • Abdominal pain	• Increase fibre intake • Exercise most days of the week • Don't ignore the urge to have a bowel movement • Laxatives

What is it?	Symptoms	Treatment
• Is loose, watery and potentially more frequent bowel movements • Most episodes are usually short-lived however if it lasts longer it could be something more serious	• Loose, watery stools • Abdominal cramps • Abdominal pain • Fever • Blood in the stool • Mucus in the stool • Bloating • Nausea • Urgent need to have a bowel movement	• Keep hydrated • Antibiotics if cause is a bacterial infection

CHOLECYSTITIS

What is it?	Symptoms	Treatment
<ul><li>Is inflammation of the gallbladder</li><li>It is caused by an obstruction of the cystic duct leading from the gallbladder to the duodenum</li><li>The gallbladder secretes bile from this duct and a blockage of this duct causes the bile to irritate the gallbladder leading to Cholecystitis</li></ul>	<ul><li>Right hypochondriac pain</li><li>Shoulder tip pain</li><li>Positive Murphy's sign</li><li>Fever</li><li>Diarrhoea</li><li>Nausea/ vomiting</li></ul>	<ul><li>Appropriate analgesia they may need a lot of it</li><li>Treat any symptoms they have</li></ul>

DIVERTICULITIS

What is it?	Symptoms	Treatment
<ul><li>Diverticula are small, bulging pouches that can from in the lining of the digestive system most commonly in the colon.</li><li>Diverticulitis is when at least one of the diverticula become inflamed and potentially infected.</li></ul>	<ul><li>Abdominal pain</li><li>Nausea/vomiting</li><li>Fever</li><li>Abdominal tenderness</li><li>Constipation</li></ul>	<ul><li>Antibiotics</li><li>Liquid diet</li><li>Surgery</li></ul>

GASTROENTERITIS

What is it?	Symptoms	Treatment
• Most cases caused by an enteric virus; may also be bacterial or protozoal • Norovirus is becoming a prevalent cause, Rotavirus still 4 times more common	• Diarrhoea • May contain blood and mucus with some infections • Vomiting • Abdominal cramping • Fever • Headache • Aching limbs	• Fluids • Dioralyte

CIRRHOSIS

What is it?	Symptoms	Treatment
• Is a late stage of scaring of the liver caused by many forms of liver diseases and conditions for example hepatitis and chronic alcoholism. • Every time the liver is damaged it tries to repair itself and in the process causes scar tissue to form and the more scar tissue that forms the harder it is for the liver to function.	• Fatigue • Loss of appetite • Hepatic encephalopathy • Nausea • Easily bruising • Oedema • Weight loss • Itchy skin • Jaundice • Ascites	• Treat the cause • Treat the complications • Liver transplant surgery

What is it?	Symptoms	Treatment

• Is the symptom of a disorder of the digestive tract
• The blood often appears in stool or vomit but isn't always visible so it may cause black or tarry
• If the bleed is severe it can be life-threatening
	• Vomiting blood
	  ○ Could be red or resemble coffee grounds
	• Black, tarry stool
	• Rectal bleeding
	• Light-headedness
	• Difficulty breathing
	• Loss of consciousness
	• Chest pain
	• Abdominal pain
	• Hypotension
	• Tachycardia
	• Reduced urination
		• Prehospital
		  ○ Fluids if hypotensive
		  ○ TXA
		  ○ Pre alert to ED
		• Hospital
		  ○ Medications
		  ○ Stop NSAIDs
		  ○ Surgery

URINARY

What is it?	Symptoms	Treatment
• Is where the kidney suddenly stop working properly, it can range from minor loss of kidney function to complete kidney failure • he kidneys become less able to filter waste products from the blood therefore dangerous levels of waste products accumulate and the bloods chemical make up becomes out of balance • It can be can be fatal if rapid treatment does not occur	• Decreased urine output • Fluid retention • Shortness of breath • Fatigue • Confusion • Nausea • Weakness • Irregular heart beat • Chest pain • Seizure • Coma	• Treat the cause • Dialysis • Medications to control potassium • Medication to control calcium • Balance fluid in the blood

What is it?	Symptoms	Treatment

Are deposits of minerals and salts along the urinary tract, kidneys and bladder	• Most are asymptomatic
	• Sudden severe pain
	  ○ Starting in loin
	  ○ Pain moves towards groin
	  ○ Most painful when stone is moving
	  ○ Pain radiates into the scrotum, labia or thigh
	  ○ Pain is constant with some periods of dull aching before it returns
	• Haematuria
	• Dysuria
	• Rigors
	• Fever
	• Urinary retention
	• Nausea/vomiting
		• Analgesia
		• Antiemetics
		• Most stones pass naturally in 1-3 weeks
		• Drink lots of fluids
		• Attempt to catch stones
		• If the stones don't pass the following may need to happen
		  ○ Extracorporeal shock wave lithotripsy
		  ○ Percutaneous nephrolithotomy
		  ○ Ureteroscopy
		  ○ Open surgery

URINARY TRACT INFECTION

What is it?	Symptoms	Treatment
• Is an infection in any part of the urinary system • Most infections involve the lower urinary tract • Females are more likely to get UTIs than males due to having a shorter urethra so the bacteria has less distance to the bladder • Presence of bacteriuria alone in over 65s does not usually indicate treatment is necessary	• Urinary frequency • Dysuria • Passing small amounts of urine • Haematuria • Foul smelling urine • Cloudy urine • Urinary incontinence • Urgency • Suprapubic/loin pain • Rigors • Nausea/vomiting • Pyrexia • Acute confusion	• Trimethoprim or nitrofurantoin is given for uncomplicated UTIs • Some patients take a low does of prophylactically • Paracetamol/ NSAIDs can be taken to relief symptoms

URINARY RETENTION

What is it?	Symptoms	Treatment
• Is a condition in which the bladder is unable to empty fully or partially • It can be related to other issues such as prostate issues and cystocele	• Inability to urinate/ frequent small urination • Lower abdominal pain • Urgency to urinate • Lower abdominal swelling • Flow changes, slow or stop start • Incontinence	• Pre hospital-appropriate analgesia to help keep the patient comfortable • Draining bladder • Catheters • Medications • Surgery • Physical therapy

MUSCULOSKELETAL

FRACTURES

Spiral fracture	Comminuted fracture	Transverse fracture
• MOI- twisting force causing an oblique angle • Union of the bone is normally good, but the angle of surfaces and muscle action can cause slippage and shortening	• MOI- direct force sometimes crush injuries • The bone is broken into more than two parts • They are unstable and difficult to treat, they can be accompanied with serve soft tissue, blood vessel and nerve damage	• MOI- Direct blow or bending force • Is a break at a right angle across the shaft of a long bone • If the bone ends hold a good position they can unite without shortening
Green stick fracture • MOI- any increased angulation • Are a very common paediatric injury caused by bending of the bone causing a break in the periosteum on one side of the bone	Fissure fracture • MOI- repetitive overuse with inadequate time to heal • A crack extending from the surface into but not through the bone	Oblique fracture • MOI- May result of a sharp blow that comes from an angle due to a fall or other trauma • Is a diagonal break across the bone • Often occurs in the long bones
Impact fracture • MOI- falling from height landing on feet • Fractures where a fragment is firmly driven into the other	Stress fracture • MOI- increasing the intensity of an activity too quickly • Are small cracks in the bone • Can happen to any bone	Avulsion fracture • MOI- common sports injury • Occurs near to where the bone attaches to tendons or ligaments

Open fracture
- MOI- severe force and trauma
- The broken bone pierces through the skin
- This is a serious and potentially life-threatening emergency

SPRAIN

What is it?	Symptoms	Treatment
A sprain is a stretching or tearing of a ligament	• Pain • Swelling • Bruising • Reduced movement	• R- Rest • I- Ice • C- Compression • E- Elevation • Over the counter pain medication like paracetamol and ibuprofen to help with pain and inflammation

STRAINS

What is it?	Symptoms	Treatment
• A strain is an injury to a muscle or tendon • Can be a minor injury from overstretching the muscles or tendons but serious injury can be caused which involves a partial or complete tear of the muscle or tendon	• Pain • Tenderness • Redness • Bruising • Reduced range of movement • Muscle spasms • Swelling • Muscle weakness	• R- Rest • I- Ice • C- Compression • E- Elevation • Over the counter pain medication like paracetamol and ibuprofen to help with pain and inflammation

BACK PAIN

What is it?	Symptoms	Treatment
Back pain is a very common symptom for people to have which can have a massive impact on the individuals life.	• Stiffness • Muscle spasms • Pain in the back or legs or feet • Pins and needles • Numbness • Weakness	• Medications • Over the counter pain relief • Muscle relaxants • Prescribed pain relief • Physiotherapy

ARTHRITIS

What is it?	Symptoms	Treatment

• Arthritis is the swelling and tenderness to one or more joints.
• This typically happens in old age
	• Pain
	• Stiffness
	• Swelling
	• Decreased range of movement
	• Redness
		• Medications
		  ○ NSAIDS
		  ○ Steroids
		• Physiotherapy
		• Surgery
		  ○ Joint repair
		  ○ Joint replacement
		  ○ Joint fusion

EAR, NOSE AND THROAT

VERTIGO

What is it?	Symptoms	Treatment
• Vertigo is the feeling that someone may experience where they feel like the you and everything around you is spinning • It can be the result of a problem in the inner ear, or the vestibular nerve can be triggered by rapid changes in head movement	• Dizziness • Loss of balance • Nausea and vomiting • A sense that you or the surroundings are moving/spinning • Nystagmus	• Epley manoeuvres and other slow-moving manoeuvres which have the goal of moving particle from the fluid filled semicircular canals into the vestibule which makes it easier for the particles to be reabsorbed • If these positionings don't help and is persistent you may be referred to ENT for surgery

TONSILLITIS

What is it?	Symptoms	Treatment
• Is the inflammation of the tonsils	• Red swollen tonsils • White or yellow patches or coating on the tonsils • Sore throat • Painful swallow • Difficulty swallowing • Fever • Enlarged lymph nodes in the neck • Bad breath • Headache • Scratchy voice • stomach-ache • Stiff neck or neck pain	• Only need antibiotics if tonsillitis is caused by an bacteria • Over the counter medications such as paracetamol • Throat lozenges may help with sore throat • Plenty of fluids • Rest

OTITIS EXTERNA

What is it?	Symptoms	Treatment
• Otitis externa also known as swimmer's ear is an infection of the outer ear canal	• Itchy ear • Redness in the ear • Discomfort of the ear that's made worse when you pull on the pinna • Fluid leaking from the ear that's odourless • Severe pain that might radiate to other areas such as face and neck • Swollen lymph nodes • Fever	• Ear drops to clean the ears if needed • Antibiotics to treat the infection this can be via drops or oral tablets • Over the counter medications such as paracetamol and ibuprofen to treat the discomfort and fever if you have any

OTITIS MEDIA

What is it?	Symptoms	Treatment
• This is an infection of the middle ear	• Ear pain • Fluid from the ear • Trouble hearing • Loss of balance • Fever • Headache • Loss of appetite	• This depends sometimes clinicians will wait and see as it may not need antibiotic treatment • Manage pain with over-the-counter pain relief such as paracetamol and ibuprofen • If needed antibiotics

ENDOCRINOLOGY

What is it?	Symptoms	Treatment
• This makes these levels of glucose in the blood to become too high. • This happened when the body cannot produce enough of a hormone called insulin's which function is to control blood sugar.	• Increased thirst • Frequent urination • Extreme hunger • Unexplained weight loss • Presence of ketones in the urine • Fatigue - Irritability • Blurred vision • Slow healing • Frequent infections	• Healthy eating • Physical activity • Monitor blood sugars • Insulin • Medications • Transplantation of pancreas

What is it?	Symptoms	Treatment
It is a condition where the insulin in the pancreas doesn't work properly, or the pancreas can't make enough insulin this means the blood glucose levels keep rising.	• Increased thirst • Frequent urination • Increased hunger • Unintended weight loss • Fatigue • Blurred vision • Slow healing • Frequent infections • Numberless or tingling in the hands or feet • Hyperpigmentation	• Healthy eating • Physical activity • Monitor blood sugars • Insulin • Medications

Diabetic ketoacidosis

What is it?	Symptoms	Treatment

• DKA is a life-threatening diabetic emergency.
• DKA is an acute metabolic complication of diabetic which is characterised by hyperglycaemia, hyperketonaemia, and metabolic acidosis. It develops when there are insufficient insulin levels for the body's basic metabolic requirements.
• Insulin deficiency causes the body to metabolise fat instead of glucose for energy. This leads to an accumulation of glucose within the blood resulting in hyperglycaemia
	• Excessive thirst
	• Frequent urination
	• Nausea and vomiting
	• Stomach pain
	• Fatigue or weak
	• Short of breath
	• Fruity-scented breath
	• Confusion
	• High blood sugar levels
	• Coma
	• Cramps
	• High ketones levels
		• Prehospital
		  ◦ Understate an ABCD assessment
		    ▪ Correct any ABC problems
		    ▪ Consider giving IV fluids if there is clear evidence of circulatory failure or dehydration
		  ◦ Is this patient being time critical fix ABCs and transfer to the nearest receiving hospital
		  ◦ Look for medical alert information
		  ◦ Assess blood glucose levels
		  ◦ Assess for signs of dehydration
		  ◦ Assess heart rhythm through an ECG
		  ◦ Measure oxygen saturations
		  ◦ Provide a pre alert to the receiving hospital
		  ◦ Keep documentation - If patient has a record of blood sugars take it with you
		• In hospital
		  ◦ Fluid replacement
		  ◦ Electrolyte replacement
		  ◦ Insulin therapy

What is it?	Symptoms	Treatment

Addison's disease also known as adrenal insufficiency is an uncommon but serious disorder that occurs when a person doesn't produce enough cortisol or aldosterone. This means that people with Addison's need to take hormone replacement to replace the hormones they don't produce	• Signs of crisis
	  ○ Severe weakness
	  ○ Confusion
	  ○ Pain in your lower back or legs
	  ○ Severe abdominal pain
	  ○ Vomiting
	  ○ Diarrhoea
	  ○ Reduced consciousness
	  ○ Delirium
	  ○ Hypotension
	  ○ Hyperkalaemia
	  ○ Hyponatremia
	• Signs of Addison's
	  ○ Hyperpigmentation
	  ○ Severe fatigue
	  ○ Unintentional weight loss
	  ○ Nausea
	  ○ Vomiting
	  ○ Abdominal pain
	  ○ Fainting
	  ○ Salt craving
	  ○ Dizziness
	  ○ Muscle and joint pain
		• Prehospital
		  ○ Hydrocortisone
		  ○ Fluids
		  ○ Transport to ED
		• Hospital
		  ○ Hormone replacement therapy

PEADIATRICS

CROUP

What is it?	Symptoms	Treatment

• Is an infection of the upper airway that caused obstructed breathing and causes a characteristic barking cough.
• The cough is a result of swelling around the larynx, trachea, and bronchi. When they cough air is forced outed out of the narrowed bronchi and through the swollen vocal cords produces a noise similar to a seal barking and when taking a breath out it often produces a high pitch whistling sound called stridor
	• Fever and coryza for 1-3 days
	• Symptoms often start or a worse at night
	• Mild fever <38.5
	• Little or no respiratory difficulty
	• Stridor depends on narrowing
	• Tachypnoea
	• Tachycardia
	• Recession
	• Hypoxia
	• Agitation
		• ABCDE approach
		• Maintain SPo2
		• Supportive treatment
		• Dependant on severity rapid transport
		• Some trusts carry dexamethasone or nebulised adrenaline to treat croup
		• In hospital treatment,
		  ○ Oral dexamethasone 150mcg/kg
		  ○ Nebulised Budesonide 2mg

FEBRILE CONVULSIONS

What is it?	Symptoms	Treatment
• Is a neurological abnormality that occurs as a result of an infection in which the immune system response by inducing a fever which raises the core body temperature. • The increase in temperature leads to an increase in neuronal excitability which results in a convulsion.	• Fever • Loss of consciousness • Shaking or jerking of the body	• Lower the patient's temperature • Keep hydrated • Treat the cause of the infection

HYPOGLYCAEMIA

What is it?	Symptoms	Treatment
• Is a condition in which the blood glucose level is lower than normal. • Very common with children who are ill	• Irregular heart rate • Tachycardia • Fatigue • Shakiness • Pale skin • Anxiety • Sweating • Hunger • Irritability • Tingling and numbness of the lips, tongue, or check • Confusion • Visual disturbance • Seizures • Loss of consciousness	• If they can eat have something sugary followed by some slow acting carbohydrates such as toast • Glucose's gel 40% can be given • Glucagon • 10% glucose given IV can be given if they are unconscious or if other treatments haven't worked

BRONCHIOLITIS

What is it?	Symptoms	Treatment

Is an inflammation of the lining of the bronchioles, causing them to become irritated and inflamed, patients to cough up thickened mucus which can be discoloured.	• Cough
	• Production of mucus
	• Fatigue
	• Shortness of breath
	• Slight fever and chills
	• Chest discomfort
		• Give oxygen if SpO2 persistently <92%
		• Do not treat with
		  ○ Antibiotic
		  ○ Adrenaline (nebulised)
		  ○ Salbutamol
		  ○ Ipratropium bromide
		  ○ Corticosteroids
		• Hospital treatment may consist of fluids, CPAP, and other supportive therapies

CHICKEN POX

What is it?	Symptoms	Treatment
Is an infection caused by the varicella-zoster virus causing an itchy rash with small fluid filled blisters. It is highly contagious and can be vaccinated against it however in the UK it is not common for this to happen as the likely hood of a young child getting seriously ill from it is minimal.	• Fever • Loss of appetite • Headache • Tiredness • Feeling unwell • Raised pink or red bumps • Small fluid filled blisters • Crusts and scabs	• Paracetamol for fever • Treat any serious complications

DEHYDRATION

What is it?	Symptoms	Treatment
This is where your body is losing more fluids than it is taking in, if not treated it can become serious.	• Dry mouth and tongue • No tears when crying • No wet nappies in 3 hours • Sunken eyes and checks • Sicken soft spot on the top of the skull • Listlessness • Irritability	• Rehydration solutions such as Dioralyte • IV fluids maybe needed

TRUAMA

NECK OF FEMUR FRACTURE

What is it?	Symptoms	Treatment

• A neck of femur fracture or NOF is a particular type of hip fracture that occurs at the femoral head.	• Pain
	• Unable to move
	• Unable to weight bear
	• Leg shortened and rotated
	• Swelling on the side of the hip
		• Prehospital
		  ○ Check for other injuries
		  ○ Immobilize the injury
		  ○ Give appropriate pain relief
		  ○ Transport to hospital
		• Hospital
		  ○ X-rays
		  ○ Usually, surgery
		  ○ Pain Management
		  ○ Rehabilitation

INTRACRANIAL BLEED

What is it?	Symptoms	Treatment

• It is a collection of blood on the brain caused by a ruptured blood vessel in the brain, this can be caused by trauma such as a car accident or a haemorrhagic stroke
• It is a potentially life-threatening issue that needs immediate hospital treatment and potential surgery
	• Increased headache
	• Vomiting
	• Drowsiness
	• Dizziness
	• Loss of consciousness
	• Confusion
	• Unequal pulses
	• Slurred speech
	• Paralysis
	• Seizures
		• Prehospital
		  ○ Make sure that you fix ABCDE problems first
		  ○ Hypotensive think about fluids
		  ○ Are they over 18 with a GCS less than 12 TXA can be given
		  ○ Pre alert to hospital, Major trauma/stroke centre depending on if available and cause
		• Hospital
		  ○ Surgery
		  ○ May wait and see if the body absorbs it

PNEUMOTHORAX

What is it?	Symptoms	Treatment
• Is a collapsed lung • Occurs when air leaks into the pleural cavity this air pouches on the outside of the lung causing the lung to collapse	• Sudden onset pain • Dyspnoea • Tachycardia • Hypotension • Hyper-resonance and reduced breath sound over the area • Decreased movement of affected side	• Needle thoracentesis • Chest drains • Surgery

HAEMOTHORAX

What is it?	Symptoms	Treatment

• Is when blood collects between the chest wall and the lung, the pleural cavity
• It can range from undetectable to life-threatening
  ○ Each side of the thorax holds 3 litres of blood
	• Chest pain
	• Cold, pale, clammy skin
	• Tachycardia
	• Hypotension
	• Tachypnoea
	• Difficulty breathing
	• Feeling restless
	• Anxiety
		• Treat for shock if present
		• Treat for blood loss
		• Rapid transport
		• Hospital
		  ○ Chest drains
		  ○ Fix the cause

MATERNITY

PLACENTA PREVIA

What is it?	Symptoms	Treatment
An abnormally sited placenta, which lies low down in the uterus and partially or wholly occluded the opening of the cervix	• Severe haemorrhage during pregnancy especially if labour has begun • Unlikely to be in pain • Blood loss is usually bright red • To begin with blood flow or the foetus is not compromised	• Pain relief • Treat the hypotension is needed • Treat the hypovolemia is needed

ECTOPIC PREGNANCY

What is it?	Symptoms	Treatment
• An ectopic pregnancy occurs when a fertilized egg implants and grows outside the main cavity of the uterus. • An ectopic pregnancy most often occurs in a fallopian tube • Sometimes, an ectopic pregnancy occurs in other areas of the body, such as the ovary, abdominal cavity, or the lower part of the uterus	• Abdominal/ pelvic pain • Amenorrhoea • Vaginal bleeding • Shoulder tip pain • Rectal pain • Gastrointestinal symptoms	• <C> ABCDE • Monitor for signs of shock • Assess volume of blood loss and consider fluids and TXA • When did they last feel the baby move • Assess Pain and treat accordingly • Depending on local and gestation take to maternity unit or ED

MISCARRIAGE

What is it?	Symptoms	Treatment
• In the UK, any pregnancy lost before 24 weeks • After 24 weeks loss of pregnancy is known as a stillbirth • Miscarriages are not registered	• Bleeding, light, heavy of tern with clots and jelly-like tissue • Pain ○ Central, crampy, suprapubic or with backache • Hypotension • Signs of pregnancy may be subsided	• <C> ABCD • Monitor for signs of shock • Assess volume of blood loss and consider fluids and TXA • When did they last feel the baby move • Assess Pain and treat accordingly • Depending on local area and gestation take to maternity unit or ED

POST PARTUM HEAMORRHAGE

What is it?	Symptoms	Treatment

• Is heavy bleeding after birth.
• They fall into 2 types, primary and secondary.
  ○ Primary post-partum haemorrhage- Is when they lose more than 500ml or more within in the first 24 hours after the birth. They can be minor is they lose 500-1000ml or major when they lose more than 1000ml in the first 24 hours.
  ○ Secondary post-partum haemorrhage- Occurs when there is abnormal or heavy vaginal bleeding between 24 hours and 12 weeks after birth.
	• Uncontrolled bleeding
	• Hypotension
	• Tachycardia
	• Decreased red blood cells
	• Swelling and pain in tissues in the vaginal and perineal area
		• Medications for the bleed
		  ○ Misoprostol, Syntometrine, TXA
		• Treat the hypotension with fluids if systolic is under 90mmhg
		• Treat shock
		• Rapid transfer to hospital

PLACENTAL ABRUPTION

What is it?	Symptoms	Treatment
• A normal sited placenta that becomes detached from the uterine wall resulting in blood loss in the retro-placental area, which causes further detachment of the placenta from the uterine wall • Blood loss can be revealed or concealed dependent on the degree of separation	• Vaginal bleeding • Abdominal pain • Back pain • Uterine tenderness or rigidity • Uterine contraction	• Pain relief • Treat the hypotension is needed • Treat the hypovolemia is needed

PREECLAMPSIA

What is it?	Symptoms	Treatment

• Is a disorder of widespread vascular endothelial malfunction and vasospasm that occurs after 20 weeks gestation and can present as late as 6 weeks post-partum.
• It is defined as by hypertension and proteinuria with or without pathological oedema
	• Protein in the urine
	• Severe headaches
	• Changes in vision
	• Upper abdominal pain
	• Nausea and vomiting
	• Decreased urine output
	• Decreased levels of platelets in the blood
	• Impaired liver function
	• Shortness of breath
		• Medications
		  ○ Medication to lower blood pressure
		  ○ Corticosteroids
		  ○ Anticonvulsant medications
		• Bed rest
		• Hospitalisation
		• Delivery of the baby

What is it?	Symptoms	Treatment
• Is a severe complication of preeclampsia • It is very rare but serious condition where high blood pressure that results in seizures during pregnancy	• Hypertension • Swelling in hands and face • Headaches • Excessive weight gain • Nausea and vomiting • Visual problems • Difficulty urinating • Abdominal pain • Seizures • Loss of consciousness • Agitation	• Medications • Delivery of baby

MENTAL HEALTH

What is it?	Symptoms	Treatment

• Anxiety is what some feels when they are worried, tense, or afraid particularly about things that have happened or are going to happen in the future
• It is a normal human response when someone feels under threat however when this is something that happens all the time this is something to be concerned about.
• It can be experienced through someone's thoughts feelings and physical sensations
	• Feeling nervous, restless, or tense
	• Having a sense of impending danger, panic, or doom
	• Having an increased heart rate
	• Breathing rapidly (hyperventilation)
	• Sweating
	• Trembling
	• Feeling weak or tired
	• Trouble concentrating or thinking about anything other than the present worry
	• Having trouble sleeping
	• Experiencing gastrointestinal (GI) problems - Having difficulty controlling worry
	• Having the urge to avoid things that trigger anxiety
		• Medication
		• Talking therapy
		• Lifestyle changes
		  o Keep physical activity
		  o Avoid drugs and alcohol
		  o Don't smoke
		  o Reduce caffeine intake
		  o Meditation
		  o Eat healthy
		  o Good sleep routine

SELF HARM

What is it?	Why does someone self-harm	Treatment
It is when someone deliberately hurts themselves examples include • Taking too many tablets-overdosing • Cutting • Burning • Banging head themselves or throwing against something hard • Punching themselves • Scratching It is a fairly common especially in those who have a mental illness	• Feeling depressed • Feeling bad about themselves • Physical or sexual abuse • Relationship problems • Hopeless • Want control their lives • Isolated	Make sure that you treat anyone with self-harm with dignity and respect Treat the act of self-harm Seek support to help stop and understand • This can be assessed through your GP • Through psych liaison team in the hospital • Through charities

DEPRESSION

What is it?	Symptoms	Treatment

• Depression is a low mood that lasts for a long time and effects a person's daily life	• Sleep disturbance
	• Change of appetite
	• Loss of interest
	• Irritability
	• Unwanted emotional outbursts
	• Anxiety
	• Difficulty concentrating
	• Lack of focus
	• Substance abuse
	• Poor hygiene
		• Medications
		• Talking therapy
		• Lifestyle
		  ○ Learn your triggers
		  ○ Avoid alcohol and drugs
		  ○ Look after yourself

What is it?	Symptoms	Treatment
• Is a condition that affects the way the brain processes information which can cause a person to lose touch with reality	Psychotic episode • Hallucinations • Auditory hallucinations- Hearing voices when no one is around • Tactile hallucinations- Strange sensations or feeling they can't explain • Visual hallucinations- Where they can see people or things that aren't there or thing that the shape of things looks wrong Delusions • Outside forces are in control of feelings and actions • Small events or comments have a huge meaning • Believe they have special powers, they on a special mission or they feel like god	• Antipsychotic medications • CBT • Social support

Hypomania	Mania
Less severe than mania that last usually for a few days Usually able to continue with day-to-day life with limited effect on their lives but people may notice a change in their mood and it being more elevated How they feel • Happy • Euphoric • Very excited • Irritable and agitated • Increased sexual energy • Easily distracted Behaviours • Being more active than normal • Talking a lot or speaking very quickly • Very friendly • Sleeping very little • Spending more money • Taking risks • Losing social inhibitions	More severe lasts at least a week Lasts for at least one week or more and has a severe negative impact on a person's ability to usual day-to-day activities Behaviours • More active than usual • Talks a lot, may not make sense • Very friendly • Saying and doing things out of character • Not sleeping or sleeping very little • Being rude or aggressive • Misusing drugs or alcohol • Spending money excessively • Losing social inhibitions • Taking serious risks with your safety How they feel • Happy • Euphoric • Uncontrollably excited • Irritable and agitated • Increased sexual energy • Easily distracted • Very confident or adventurous • Feel untouchable or can't be harmed • Feel that they can perform task better than normal • See or hear things that other people can't

Printed in Great Britain
by Amazon

22170640R00041